A Guide to Burn Ca

• Recovery • First Aid • Prevention

Written by Kenneth Wright
In consultation with Judy Knighton, R.N., M.Sc.N.; from the
Sunnybrook Hospital, Ross Tilley Burn Centre, Toronto

Thanks also to: Maryann Smith, B.A., R.N.; Jane TenEycke,
B.Sc., R.N.; Bonnie Abdale, M.S.W.; Sylvia Cooper, B.Sc., O.T;
Lydia Pashutiniski, B.A.Sc., R.P.D.T, and Evelyn Paul, R.P.T.

Acknowledgement for information provided by St. John
Ambulance and The Red Cross. Also our thanks to the editing
work from the nurse members of the WOCN and the many
surveys completed from Burn Centers in North America.

Burn care. Burn prevention. Burn first aid. Self help.
Burn recovery.

ISBN # 978 1 896616 12 4

Printed in U.S.A.

Glossary

Antimicrobial: A substance that will kill or stop the growth of microorganisms like bacteria.

Contractures: Restricted movement of a joint caused by scar tissue or loss of normal stretchiness of the skin.

CPR – Cardiopulmonary Resuscitation: A first aid technique for reviving a patient who is unconscious, not breathing and pulseless.

Debridement: Removal of dirt and dead tissue from a burn wound.

Epithelialization: The regrowth of skin cells.

Eschar: The scab or dry crust of a burn wound.

Grafting: Skin tissue taken from a site or a person and put into a new site or person.

Hydrotherapy: The use of water to treat physical problems.

Hypertrophy: An increase in the size of the skin caused by an increase in the size of the skin cells rather than the number of cells.

Necrotic: Pertaining to dead skin tissue.

ROM: Exercises that will improve the Range of Motion of joints.

Superficial: Relating to the top surface of the skin.

Topical: Referring to the surface of a part of the body.

Tubbing: The name for a specialized bath as part of burn treatment.

Table of Contents

Introduction

Burn care and subsequent healing is probably not a topic that the average person would read about if given the choice between a good book or magazine article. However, burn accidents do happen, and survivors, caregivers and family members have to deal with the uphill battle of recovery and returning to a normal quality of life.

The pain, discomfort and amount of time it takes to recover from this sort of injury makes for a traumatic experience for everyone concerned.

In North America, almost 2.5 million burns are treated in hospitals each year – most of these could have been prevented. We hope this book can help to greatly reduce that number by creating awareness of the traumatic nature of burn injuries and providing some simple common sense measures that can be taken to prevent them.

With this in mind, we like to think the purposes of this book are as follows:

A. To create awareness of the nature and seriousness of burns.

B. To motivate the reader to take all possible preventive and safety actions at home or at work in order to avoid such an accident on your part or that of a family member.

C. To provide information on what to do if a fire breaks out in your home.

D. To enable the reader to give basic first aid to someone suffering from a burn injury.

E. To remove any fears and concerns you may have about burn treatment.

The information in this book is basic, and does not involve any "hands-on" training or role playing. Consequently, we suggest that if you wish to be truly competent and confident when it comes to first aid, you should enroll in a local community training class or St. John Ambulance course. This is especially relevant for the more complex artificial respiration and cardio resuscitation instructions for electrical burn injuries.

It is very important to comply with treatment and follow the procedures for caring for a burn "to the letter" to ensure the best possible outcome for you or your loved one.

This book is not meant to replace the advice of your physician or nurse regarding burn care or treatment. If anything, the material here is designed to help you communicate with your health care team in order to improve your success and satisfaction with your treatment.

Section 1:
Understanding Burns
and First Aid

Types of burns

There are four major types of burns, depending on the nature of the accident:

1. Thermal burns

There are usually two categories of thermal burns:

- Skin injury from dry heat due to contact with a flame or hot object. Usually a large surface area of the body is affected and the burn damage may be quite deep into the skin.
- Scalds caused by steam or boiling hot liquids. These types of burns range in severity from superficial to very deep and can be extremely serious if a large surface area of the body is involved.

2. Chemical burns

These are caused by strong chemicals such as acids or alkalis and can very quickly cause skin damage. They can be even more serious if these chemicals are swallowed and damage is done to the mouth and throat, or if the patient is exposed to the chemical for a prolonged period of time and absorption occurs.

3. Electrical burns

An electrical current can create a burn injury at those points where it enters and leaves the body. The burn injury in these cases can be quite deep into the skin. There are further associ-

ated problems where an electric shock can cause breathing difficulties and affect the activity of the heart. Immediate resuscitation by trained first aid or health care professionals is sometimes
necessary to save the injured person.

4. Radiation

The all-too-common problem of sunburn fits into this category;
too much exposure to the sun can cause redness, swelling and
blistering. Other sources of this sort of burn include overex-
posure to ultraviolet radiation, such as sun lamps and tanning
beds.

First aid treatment
The basic aims of burn first aid are:
1. To lesson the effects of heat.
2. To reduce pain.
3. To prevent infection of the burned skin area.

The first action to take for a severe burn or scald is to call 911 for an ambulance and any other number that can quickly bring medical help. The severity of a burn can be minimized when appropriate first aid measures are taken at the scene of the accident. The correct sequence of events immediately following a burn injury is suggested by the catch phrase, "Stop, drop, roll and cool": **Stop** – don't run; **drop** to the ground; **roll**, to put out the fire, and **cool** with water to stop the burning.

The following are general first aid tips for all burns:

Do not touch burns – this can cause infection.

Do not break blisters if they are small, look clean and are not around joints. If they do break, carefully cut away the loose skin with a clean pair of scissors and cover the open area with a clean bandage or dressing or a moist cloth until medical care is given.

Do not apply ointments, lotions, or oily dressings; they can have the effect of keeping heat in instead of letting the heat out. NO BUTTER, FLOUR OR TOOTHPASTE, PLEASE.

Do not use gauze, cotton, wool or anything likely to stick when covering a burn.

Do not give anything by mouth to an unconscious person. A person who is conscious and complains of thirst should be given small sips of water only.

Swelling can occur around the burned area, so ensure that anything constrictive – clothing, jewelry, etc. – is removed or loosened as soon as possible.

For large surface area superficial burns, seek medical help.

For all deep burns and electrical burns, seek medical help.

For burns to elderly people or infants, seek medical help.

The following first aid instructions are recommended for the different categories of burns:

Thermal burns
1. Cool the affected burn area with cold water. This can be achieved by placing it under running water, immersing it in water or by applying a wet cloth to the burn.
2. Remove rings, bracelets or other jewelry as quickly as possible before the swelling begins.
3. Cover the burn with a clean cloth or preferably a sterile, lint-free dressing (even a facial tissue will work) and secure this lightly with a bandage or one that is improvised from an article of clothing.
4. Seek hospital treatment for burns and scalds larger than the size of a quarter in area. If you have any doubts, err on the side of caution and go to the hospital.
5. Do not breathe or cough on the burn.
6. Do not touch the burn.
7. Do not break blisters.
8. Do not remove clothing stuck to a burn.
9. Do not apply medications, ointments or greasy substances to the burn.

Chemical burns
A. Wet chemicals
Corrosive chemicals such as acids and alkalis are always serious because the chemicals will continue to burn the skin for as long as they remain there.
1. Immediately flush the chemical away with water – lots of water!
2. Do not wait to remove clothing around the affected area.
3. Continue flooding the affected area while removing clothing at the same time.

4. Continue flooding until all the corrosive chemical has been washed away.
5. Do not use any so-called chemical neutralizers such as vinegar, baking soda or alcohol to treat any chemical burns.
6. If a corrosive chemical spills on the eye, flush the eye slowly with running water for at least 10 minutes. If necessary, hold the eyelids open with your fingers.
7. Continue the first aid instructions as previously described for a thermal burn from points 2 to 9.

B. Dry chemicals
If the chemical is not wet but dry – like lime, a common corrosive – it should be brushed off before flushing or flooding the burn injury with water. Then, follow all the instructions listed for first aid treatment of a wet corrosive chemical.

Electrical burns
Burns from this type of injury may be far more serious than they appear. There could be life-threatening associated injuries involving breathing or heart difficulties. The injured person may have been violently thrown by the force of the electrical shock, causing serious physical injuries such as broken bones or damage to internal organs. It is vital in these cases to seek emergency medical assistance.
1. Do not touch the injured person until the electricity is turned off.
2. Carefully turn off the electrical source causing the injury.
3. Check the injured person for pulse and breathing.
4. Give artificial respiration or cardiopulmonary resuscitation (CPR) if necessary (see instructions on the following pages).
5. Locate the burn damage area. This is usually located where the electrical current entered and left the body.
6. Apply a clean, dry dressing over the burn areas.
7. If you have not already done so, seek medical aid by calling 911 or other means.

Artificial Respiration Guidelines

Adult Casualty
A. Give two breaths
1. Open the airway.
2. Cover the casualty's mouth with your own and pinch nostrils (fig 1).
3. Give enough air to make the chest rise.

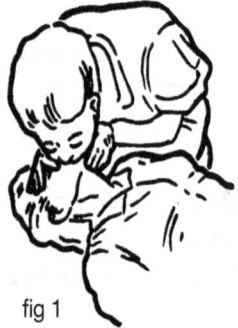

fig 1

B. Check for carotid pulse for 5-10 seconds (fig 2)
1. If pulse present, give one breath every 5 seconds.
2. If pulse absent, START cardio-pulmonary resuscitation (CPR).

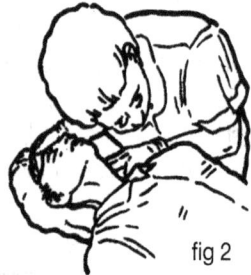

fig 2

Child Casualty
A. Give two breaths
1. Open the airway.
2. Cover the child's mouth with your mouth and pinch the nostrils.(fig 3)
3. Just give enough air to make the chest rise.

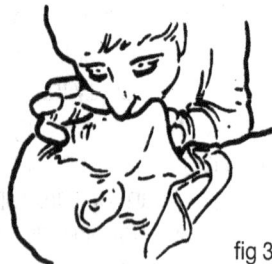

fig 3

B. Check carotid pulse for 5 - 10 seconds
1. If pulse present give one breath every 3 seconds. (fig 4)
2. If pulse absent START CPR.

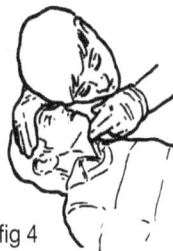

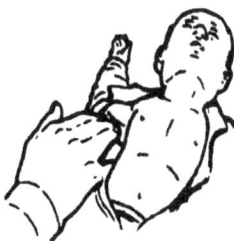

fig 4

Infant Casualty
A. Give two breaths
1. Open the airway.
2. Cover the infant's mouth and nose with your mouth (fig 5).
3. Give just enough air to make the chest rise.

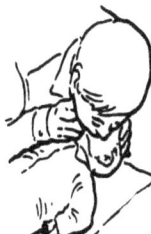

fig 5

B. Check brachial artery (inside upper arm) pulse for 5 - 10 seconds (fig 6)
1. If pulse present give one breath every 3 seconds.
2. If pulse absent, START CPR.

fig 6

Cardio Pulmonary Resuscitation
Perform CPR ONLY if the casualty is:
A. UNCONSCIOUS
B. NOT BREATHING
C. PULSELESS

Adult Cpr

A. Do CPR compressions (fig 7)

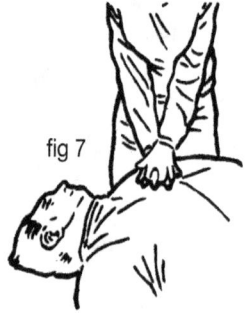
fig 7

1. Place heel of one hand on lower half on breastbone in centre of chest.
2. Place heel of other hand on top of first hand.
3. Press straight down to compress chest 1.5" - 2" (3.8 -5.0cms)
4. Press at the rate of 15 compressions in 9 seconds.

A. Give 2 breaths every 15 seconds

B. Recheck pulse and breathing after one minute.(Fig 8)

C. If pulse is still absent continue CPR until help arrives.

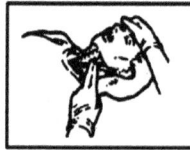
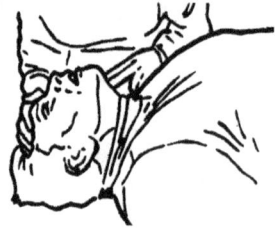
fig 8

Child Cpr
A. Do CPR compressions (Fig 9)

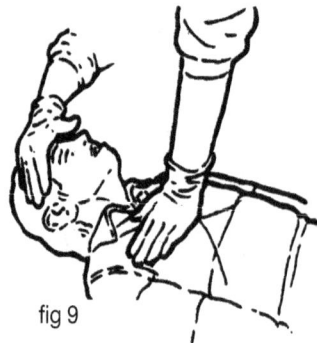
fig 9

1. Tilt back forehead with heel of one hand.
2. Place heel of other hand on lower half of breastbone in centre of the chest.
3. Press straight down to compress the chest 1 - 1.5" (2.8 - 3.8cms)
4. Press at the rate of 5 compressions every 3 seconds .

B. Give one breath after every 5 compressions.

C. Recheck pulse and breathing after one minute of CPR (fig 10).

D. If pulse still absent continue compression until help arrives.

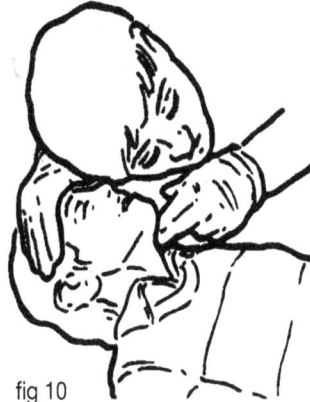

fig 10

Infant Cpr

A. Do CPR compressions (fig 11)

1. Tilt back forehead with the heel of one hand.

2. Place two fingers of the other hand in the centre of the chest, one finger width below nipple line.

3. Press straight down to compress chest ½ - 1".

4. Press at the rate of 5 compressions every 3 seconds or less.

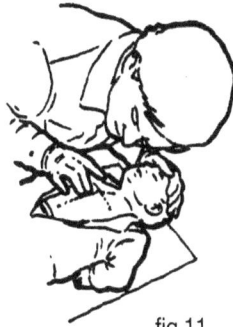

fig 11

B. Give one breath after every 5 compressions

C. Recheck pulse and breathing after one minute of CPR. (fig 12)

D. If pulse is still absent continue compressions until help arrives.

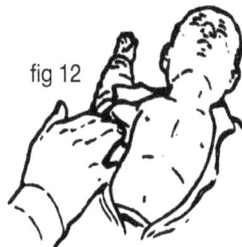

fig 12

Radiation burns
There is no specific first aid treatment for radiation burns. However, minor sunburn can be treated as follows:
Wet a towel with tap water and squeeze out the excess water
Cover the burned area with this wet towel. This will soothe and cool the skin.
Only use ointments and creams recommended by a health care professional.

Assessing the burn
The medical team will objectively assess the injury with regard to initial treatment and long term care. However, in order to understand the devastation a burn can cause, it is important to appreciate the role our skin plays in our physical well-being.
Our skin performs the following functions:
1. Protects the body from infection
2. Controls body temperature
3. Retains body fluids.

The severity of a burn depends upon:
1. The amount of body surface affected
2. The location of the burn – around the face or throat could be considered critical since it might affect breathing
3. The depth of the injury
4. The age of the patient and his or her general state of health.

The categories of burn depth are usually described as follows:
1. Superficial partial-thickness burns, also known as mild second-degree burns. These burns and scalds affect the shallow outer layers of the skin. They resemble sunburns and can be very painful, but will usually heal within 10 days.

2. Deep partial-thickness burns, also known as deep second-degree burns. These can be very painful; blisters can form and the injury takes 14 to 21 days to heal.

3. Full-thickness burns, also known as third-degree burns. These involve damage to all layers of the skin including the skin-reproducing cells. The skin will require skin grafting in order for the burn injury to heal.

The two generalized types of burns can be summarized as follows:

1. The burned area is reddish, swollen and may blister. The pain can initially be severe, but the healing is rapid and leaves little scarring.

2. Deep burns are those in which the whole thickness of the skin is affected. There is usually less pain initially because the nerve endings may have been temporarily destroyed. Healing can be slow and scars may develop.

It is not always possible for the medical team to tell the severity of the injury at the time of diagnosis. It often takes several days to find out whether the burn wound will heal on its own or whether grafting is needed. Consequently, it follows that it is not always possible to predict exactly how long it will take for a burn injury to completely heal.

Section 2:
Medical Treatment of the Burn

When you have a burn injury, you may be sent to the emergency department of your local hospital. Here, your burn injury will be assessed and treatment begun. The physician at the hospital may decide you would benefit from being treated at a more specialized facility called a burn center. Therefore, you may be transferred to a different department or to another hospital where the burn centre is located.

These burn centres are usually small units containing around 10 beds. They are comprehensively equipped to effectively treat patients with critical burn injuries. Health care professionals at these centres are highly trained and experienced, each with a different key role to help you recover from your injury and are made as comfortable as possible. They have an unusual degree of empathy to help patients through the difficult emotional trauma associated with severe burn injuries.

The burn team

In case you wish to compile a list of questions for the various specialists at a burn centre, here are the various members of the burn team. We have provided space to for you to write down any questions you may have:

Physicians

Primarily, plastic surgeons oversee all the care given to patients at a burn centre. As the burn injury heals, these medical specialists have the expertise to ensure the best possible healing and the least amount of scarring. Other medical specialists may be called on under the guidance of the plastic surgeon. You may hear the term "fellow" or "resident"; these are qualified physicians training to become specialists in burn care. They have been assigned to the burn unit under the supervision of the plastic surgeon.

Questions to ask the physician:

....
....
....
....
....
....
....
....

Nursing staff

The nurses who work in the burn centre are the mainstay of all patient care in the unit. Because of the nature of burn injuries, these nurses work with patients for long periods of time and get to know them and their families very well.

The role of the nurse is to offer as much supportive care as possible and ensure the patients' critical needs are communicated to the appropriate members of the burn team. The degree of emotional support, positive mental outlook and caring that these nurses provide to patients and family members is very important to the patients' overall recovery.

Nurses assess, on an ongoing basis, the patient's condition and assist the physician in the planning and implementation of treatment.

There may also be a clinical nurse specialist who works directly with patients and family members, providing teaching and psychological support in the burn centre and the hospital, as well as after the patient is discharged from the medical facility. Such a nurse works with the bedside nurse and the other members of the medical team on all patient care issues.

The administrator of the burn centre's nursing unit is responsible for coordinating all aspects of patient care, ensuring all the necessary resources (products, personnel, equipment and so on) are available. This nurse is in charge of the management and smooth running of the burn centre.

While patients and family members will probably have contact with all the various nursing specialists mentioned above, the initial key nurse to speak with about the daily issues of care is the bedside nurse on duty that day.

Questions to ask the bedside nurse:

....
....
....
....
....
....
....
....
....
....
....

Dietician

A burn injury makes huge demands on the body and there is usually a basic need for a well balanced, high protein, high calorie diet to ensure the healing nutritional requirements are met. Patients generally need a variety of extra supplements, vitamins and minerals that the dietician can order. After discharge from the medical facility, patients must keep to a sound nutritional plan to maintain optimum healing.

Questions to ask the dietician:

....
....
....
....
....
....
....
....
....
....
....

Physiotherapist

Also known as the physical therapist, this health care professional helps patients regain or maintain physical functioning, like arm or leg movement, that may have been diminished after the burn injury. The physiotherapist provides patients with a range of motion (ROM) exercises that, over a period of time, help get the muscles and joints back to normal. Initially, these exercises are generally carried out in the hydrotherapy room or when the dressings are removed. In this way, the exercises will not be restricted due to bulky dressings. In most cases, it is important to begin the exercises as soon as possible.

Questions to ask the physiotherapist:

....
....
....
....
....
....

Occupational therapist (OT)

These rehabilitation specialists help patients become more adaptable and self-sufficient in their daily functioning. Assistance can be provided with dexterity exercises or adaptive devices such as special cutlery or lifting aids to help in daily activities.

Questions to ask the OT:

....
....
....
....
....
....
....
....
....

Social worker

These professionals have a comprehensive understanding of the practical and emotional issues involved with a brain injury. They are available to patients and their family members to help with the following:

- Emotional issues
- Insurance claims
- Financial assistance issues
- Accommodation issues for family members planning to stay near the burn centre
- Communication with the medical team, if necessary

Questions to ask the social worker:

....
....
....
....
....
....
....
....
....
....
....

Being an out-patient

Once you have been admitted to hospital and the initial assessment and treatment have been carried out, you may be a candidate for treatment as an out-patient. The medical team may have decided that your burns are superficial with the potential to heal by re-epithelialization (new skin cells growing on their own) within 7 to 10 days. There are other factors, such as whether you live nearby and the support – or lack of support – you have at home; whether the burns are located in non-critical parts of the body, and whether you are capable of participating in home treatment. These are just some of the factors the medical team will take into consideration when making its assessment. As an out-patient, you may be required to come to the hospital every day or every three days – each case is unique.

Treatment

Upon arrival at the burn centre or emergency department, the first priority is to ensure that the patient's breathing airway is open and that lost bodily fluids are replaced. After this, the severity of the burn is determined and treatment priorities are established. Burn severity is assessed according to the following five factors:

1. The extent of the burn;
2. The depth of the burn wound;
3. The age of the injured person;
4. The patient's medical history, and
5. The part of the body that is burned.

The actual choice of treatment can vary, but all burn centres have the same common objectives:

Prevention of infection or desiccation (drying out) of the wound
- Removal of unnecessary tissue
- Preparation of a clean wound bed for new skin to grow
- Healing of skin grafts
- Minimization of systemic (within the body) infection
- Reduction of scars and contractures

In the beginning, a burn injury carries with it a sense of emergency due to pain and the necessity to minimize the initial skin damage. Burn centres and emergency departments are aware of the necessary priorities of care. The emergent period, for instance, is the time during which all the activities take place when you initially arrive at the medical facility. Following this is the acute period, where the focus is on wound care and prevention/management of any complications. The third or rehabilitation phase focuses on restoring the patient to a productive place in society.

The following is an overview of the many different treatments a patient can experience:

Burn bath or shower, also known as hydrotherapy

The patient may be immersed in a burn bath or showered on a cart shower, where initial cleansing and assessment of the burn takes place. These baths may be carried out once a day or periodically throughout the hospital stay until the wounds are healed.

The bath is usually a saline-water bath; alternatively, the patient may be gently showered with tap water while lying on a plinth. During this hydrotherapy, loose dead tissue (known as eschar) can be gently removed (debrided) using sterile scissors and forceps. Pain medication should always be given and the treatment limited to about 20 minutes or up until the point where the patient can't tolerate the treatment for long.

After this burn bath or shower, further decisions are made regarding how to treat the wound.

Cleansing the wound

Gentle, but thorough, cleansing of the burn areas with soft gauze can remove some of the sot and loose debris for easier inspection of the wound. Chemical burns will be flushed or flooded with water for 20 minutes or longer. Tar burns require numerous applications of emulsifying agents, such as Tween 80®, or Polysporin® ointment, or vegetable or mineral oil. After several days, it will be possible to remove the tar without damaging any of the healthy tissue.

Here is a basic scenario of treatment for a variety of burns:

Minor Burn Wounds

Body Burns

Layer	Dressing	Rationale
Inner	Petroleum gauze e.g. jelonet	Protects re epithelizing tissue
Middle	normal saline	Prevents drying out
Outer	dry gauze	Promotes wicking of exudate from inner to middle layers: Protects wounds

Gauze wrap e.g. Kling holds dressing in place

Facial Burns

Layer	Dressing	Rationale
	Normal saline soaked gauze pads applied directly to burn, left on for approximately 10 minutes twice daily.	Removes exudate from face.
	Polysporin ® ointment applied to face twice daily as needed.	Prevents infection to the wound.

Major Burn Wounds

Early admission

Layer	Dressing	Rationale
Inner	Flamazine	Provides topical antimicrobial coverage.
Middle	normal saline soaked gauze.	Prevents drying out of the wound.
Outer	dry gauze	Promotes wicking of exudate from inner and middle layers.

Gauze wrap e.g. Kling holds dressing in place

Major Burn Wounds

Skin grafted ares

Layer	Dressing	Rationale
Inner	Petroleum gauze	Protect re-epithelization tissue.
Middle	normal saline soaked gauze.	Prevents drying out of the wound.
Outer	dry gauze	Promotes wicking of exudate.

Gauze wrap e.g. Kling holds dressing in place

Facial burns

Layer	Dressing	Rationale
	Normal saline soaked gauze pads applied directly to burns and left for 10 minutes twice daily.	Removes exudate from the face.
	Polysporin ® ointment applied to face daily as needed.	Prevents infection of wound.

Gauze wrap e.g. Kling holds dressing in place

Caring strategy for burn wounds

The medical team will decide upon one of three different approaches to treating the burn wound:

1. Open method
   The wound remains exposed, with only a thin layer (2mm to 4mm) of topical antimicrobial ointment spread on the burn wound surface using a sterile glove or applicator.
2. Closed method
   The dressing is left intact for two to seven days.
3. Multiple dressing changes
   The dressing is changed once or twice daily, according to an agreed-upon schedule. The frequency of changing depends upon the nature of the dressing and the condition of the wound – more or less frequency may be indicated.

Ointment or cream (topical) coverage of the burn

There are a variety of creams or topical applications that are used on the burn area at different stages of the healing process. At the beginning, it is usual to apply an antimicrobial cream whose chemical name is silver sulphadiazine. This cream protects the burn against developing an infection, which can dramatically slow down the healing process. The cream is applied on a wet dressing and covered with a dry dressing and roller wrap.

When choosing a cream or ointment, the medical team will consider the following:

a. How well it works (clinical efficacy)

b. How many types of bacteria it will kill

c. Ease of use

d. Consideration of any toxic/absorption issues

e. Its proven record in not creating difficult infections, called super-infections

f. Acceptance by patient and staff

Here is a list of some of the names of topical agents commonly used during the healing process: Flamazine, Sulfamylon® (Mafenide acetate), silver nitrate (0.5%), Furacin® (nitrofurazone), Garamycin® (gentamycin sulfate), Bacitracin with Polymyxin B (Polysporin), normal saline (0.9%), acetic acid (0.5%), and hydrogen peroxide (half strength).

Applying dressings

Following the burn bath or shower, dressings are usually applied over the burn area, with the exception of the face.

Dressings are a vital part of burn care and the healing process. Their primary role is to keep the wound clean and moist and to quicken the removal of dead skin. There are many innovative and technically advanced dressings now available from manufacturers; individual medical facilities have their own particular strategies and choices.

The following factors are considered when choosing dressings:

a. Ability to promote healing
b. Effectiveness in helping to lessen pain
c. Effectiveness in helping the debriding process
d. The amount of pressure it confers
e. Its function as an immobilizer
f. Whether or not it helps to preserve the wound site
g. Acceptance by the patient
h. The condition of the burn wound
i. The desired clinical results
j. The unique properties of the dressing and its cost

The bottom line when considering all these factors is the ultimate healing of the wound. During the healing process, the medical team can adjust their tactics and strategies according to the progress and needs of the burn, which is the number one priority.

Infection control

The prevention of infection in the burn wound is very important, and strategies are in place to reduce its occurrence. Everyone is encouraged to take the following precautions:

- extremely thorough hand washing;
- when wounds are exposed, isolation gowns, head covers and masks are worn;
- clean gloves are required for removal of soiled dressings and sterile gloves for cleansing of burn wounds and application of clean dressings or topical agents to a burn area.

Other preventive measures include:

- live plants and flowers are not permitted in the burn unit
- culture swabs are taken from patients periodically and analyzed by the laboratory;
- cubicle isolation techniques are observed in patients' rooms;
- housekeeping staff keep to specific procedures and cleanliness standards when in the burn unit, and
- plastic liners are used for hydrotherapy equipment and changed for each patient.

Intravenous replacement fluid therapy

A vital part of the body's response to a burn injury is to direct fluid out of the bloodstream and into the tissues surrounding the burn area, causing swelling around the burn area. This swelling, which decreases over time, is also known as edema; it may be present around the arms, legs and face for several days after the burn injury occurs. It is necessary to replace this lost fluid from the bloodstream with an intravenous (IV) drip. To determine how much IV fluid the patient needs, his urine output is measured and his vital signs are monitored.

Nasogastric (NG) tube

Initially, after a burn injury, the stomach may stop digesting food. Consequently, it may be necessary to insert a nasogastric (NG) tube through the patient's nose into her stomach. As soon as the stomach resumes functioning, a high calorie, high protein drink will be fed through this tube. This feeding continues until the patient is able to feed herself independently.

Breathing help

If, during the burn accident, there has been inhalation of smoke or the neck has been burned and is now swollen, the patient may have problems breathing. To ensure breathing takes place, a tube can be placed through the patient's nose or mouth and connected to the lungs. This tube is then attached to a machine called a ventilator, which will help the patient breathe properly.

Diet

Proper nutrition is vital for the healing process. Usually a high protein, high calorie intake is prescribed. All the food eaten by a patient is recorded by the nurse on a calorie count sheet. This allows the dietician to know how much food the patient is eating and if it is enough each day to ensure the healing process can take place. Family members are encouraged to bring the patient's favourite foods into the hospital on a regular basis.

Skin grafts

If the burn wound is "full thickness" – all the tissues have been destroyed – then it must be covered with healthy skin from an unburned area of the body. This is called a skin graft. The area from where the healthy skin is removed is called the donor site. After this skin graft has been taken, or harvested, the donor site is covered with a dressing. This area of skin usually heals within seven to ten days.

Before the new skin can be applied, the dead tissue must be removed from the burn area. The removal of this skin or dead tissue is called debridement or excision. This process is carried out in the operating room because strict sterile conditions are needed. The actual skin grafting may be carried performed at the same time, or it may be delayed a day or two. The donor skin can actually be stored safely in a refrigerator and then applied to the patient a few days later in the patient's room.

Most donor skin is "meshed" so that it can expand to cover a larger surface area. When healed, the grafted skin may have a sort of checkered appearance, which will gradually fade over time.

Once a skin graft is applied, the dressing will not be changed for five days. This is because it is vital not to disturb the new skin area. In fact, grafted arms and legs are often kept still by being put into a cast, splint, pins or traction. The process is so delicate that even with these precautions, re-grafting may be necessary. Healing times vary from one individual to the next, so the medical team constantly evaluates progress at each dressing change.

Pain management

Burn care and pain are normally synonymous and both the burn team and the patient should maintain an open dialogue for monitoring this critical aspect of treatment. As a patient, you should never be afraid or reluctant to communicate about any pain you may be feeling. In addition, the burn team should regularly ask how you are feeling with regard to pain. Alleviation of pain and how it contributes to a positive mental attitude in coping with the healing process is a critical factor that deserves priority status.

Medication is very effective in controlling pain and additional doses should be given before dressing changes and physiotherapy sessions.

Going home

Once you are ready to be discharged from the hospital, the most intensive and critical part of your treatment is over. However, this is just one battle won – the war is not over yet. Through education, training and communication, the burn team has empowered you to care for your skin and participate in treatment programs in order for you to have the best possible outcome after your burn injury.

You may be required to visit the hospital on an out-patient basis, depending on the nature of your injury. You may even have your dressings changed at the hospital. Conversely, you may visit your family physician in your community and see the burn team periodically.

Continuing pain management

One area which you should consider as you leave the hospital is the issue of controlling pain as you recover from your burn injury. In fact, you may experience some discomfort over the next year or two as your burn scars mature. This can be frustrating but, over time, it will improve.

While there is no absolute way to remove the discomfort, you can discuss with your physician the best approach to taking pain medications and whether or not stronger medication is needed. Here are some suggestions that may help you cope with the discomfort:

Try relaxation techniques such as deep breathing, muscle relaxation, yoga, massage therapy, meditation and so on. We are all unique in terms of what makes us relax and distracts us from feelings of discomfort. Read up on these techniques and experiment until you find what works best for you.

Walking and getting out into the fresh air can be invigorating.

Follow all skin care instructions deliberately and thoroughly; this will help quicken your recovery.

Do things you enjoy – hobbies, social events and so on. Try to get back to your previous routines. This will make you feel good and distract you from feelings of discomfort.

The ABC's of when to seek medical attention

A. Pain increases
B. Redness or red streaking appears around the wound
C. Fever of 38.9° (102° F) develops and persists for more than 18 hours.

Questions to ask before leaving the hospital:

....

....

....

....

....

....

....

....

....

....

Section 3:
Leaving the Hospital

Every burn survivor leaving a hospital has a unique set of needs, follow-up procedures and post-hospital care activities to ensure complete healing. Be sure to study all the instructions, ask questions (that you have written in this book), and be sure you know the name of the contact person at the hospital and the names and phone numbers of the support professionals you'll be dealing with.

As previously highlighted, support staff could be the physical therapist, the social worker, or the occupational therapist, to name a few. There is another key health care professional who may play an important role in your rehabilitation, and that is the home care nurse. These nurses come to your home, change your dressing and ensure your recovery is proceeding well at home.

You will probably be given an appointment to return to the burn clinic in a week or two to see the team. These appointments are extremely important to your overall recovery; if you are unable to attend, you should quickly reschedule. You should also see your family physician in order to keep him or her informed of your progress.

In many communities, there are support groups of people who have experienced the same sort of burn injury as you and can provide assistance to help you on the road to recovery. Speak to the burn team about this aspect of care.

Emotional recovery

It is completely normal to experience a wide range of emotions after leaving the hospital. You have experienced a traumatic event. You have probably felt some insecurity and anxiety about possible disfigurement and may be concerned about your physical appearance. Whether or not you have had skin grafts, a burn injury is physically debilitating. You will find yourself lacking in energy and will experience frustration at your possible loss of mobility.

All these factors can lead to anger and depression; this can affect your willingness to cooperate with your health care team, which in turn can affect your achievement of a full recovery.

Remind yourself that the worst is over – you have survived, and you owe it to yourself to resume as many of your pre-burn activities as you can. Feel free to speak to the burn team as it is quite common to feel a little depressed or sad. Help is available – you are not alone in this journey.

Be kind to yourself, give yourself time to adjust, set reasonable goals and try not to have high expectations in the short term: patience is the order of the day in this sort of rehabilitation. Think two years for full recovery; if you feel better sooner than that, then that is a bonus.

One major concern you may experience upon your return home is the reaction of family and friends to your accident. You can be sure they want to help and they probably feel as much or more anxiety as you do. The key here is communication. Take a proactive approach – discuss with them your concerns about what they may be feeling and what you're feeling as well. Once dialogue is begun, you will be amazed at how quickly a constructive and supportive climate of cooperation and love is created. Feel free to talk to the burn team about this – they can help.

One critical factor in the short term is getting enough sleep. Your regular sleep patterns will have been dramatically disrupted due to the burn injury and it may take some time to adapt. Here are some suggestions that may help:

- Avoid long naps during the day.
- Try walking outside in the fresh air with some light exercise.
- Try a relaxing activity which suits you before going to bed.
- Make sure you follow your skin care instructions to reduce itchiness.
- Keep on top of your comfort levels by optimum usage of pain medication.

Finally, remember that the burn team understands the emotional challenges that can occur after leaving the hospital and are always available to help. If you are having flashbacks or nightmares, speak to the burn team. Ask for advice on relaxation techniques and know that these flashbacks usually decrease in frequency fairly quickly and are very normal, however unsettling they might be.

Skin care

Skin care is a very important part of your rehabilitation program. Simply put, your skin needs extra attention. Here are the areas you should be attentive to:

Bathing

Naturally, it's important to keep your skin clean. Once a day, you should bathe or shower using a soft, soapy cloth to gently remove dried skin and ointments.

Other tips include:

• Avoid rubbing your skin hard when bathing or showering because this can cause your still-fragile skin to break down.

• Pat yourself dry with a soft towel.

• Use lukewarm, not hot, water.

• Consider adding a few drops of bath oil to the bath water to help moisturize your skin, but be careful not to slip in the tub.

• If your skin is very dry, do not soak in the bath. Choose to shower instead.

• Always moisturize your skin after a bath or shower with your recommended moisturizing product and, perhaps, more often throughout the day.

Moisturizing skin

It is vital to keep healed burn/grafted skin supple and moist. After a burn injury, the skin's glands are not able to produce the same amount of lubricating oils as before. Your skin may feel tight and less supple, and may be dry and scaly in appearance. Consequently, until your skin is able to produce enough of its own oil, you will have to use moisturizing products to lubricate your skin.

Choosing a moisturizing lotion

Most skin care and burn care experts recommend mild, non-perfumed, non-irritating, water-based lotions. These products will make your skin feel more supple and provide you with greater comfort. There are a few excellent products available at pharmacies with therapeutic effects that are equally good, but you may prefer one over another. Experiment with different products; talk to your pharmacist and try the ones recommended by the burn team.

Two recommended products are Smith & Nephew's Professional Care® Lotion and Schering-Plough's Complex 15® Therapeutic Moisturizing Lotion.

Avoid Vaseline® and mineral or lanolin oil-based products. These tend to clog the skin's pores and are not effectively absorbed into the deeper layers where the dryness problems begin.

Applying moisturizing lotion

Gentle massage not only increases the pliability of the skin but decreases the sensitivity of the healed skin and scar tissue.

Instructions:

1. Massage the lotion gently onto your skin with light stroking motions so as not to cause friction.
2. As time progresses and your skin becomes less fragile, you can massage more firmly.
3. Lotions should be applied as often as is necessary.
4. The amount applied should be enough to be absorbed by the skin without forming any greasy build-up. If oil is allowed to accumulate, you may notice small pimples or whiteheads forming on your skin.

Avoid itching of the skin

A healing burn injury is usually dry compared to normal skin and there may be areas of unsettled scarring. These two factors can cause itching. The problem of itching is related to the damage scratching can do to the skin. Breaking the integrity of the skin can slow down the healing process, cause possible infection and make scarring worse. Eventually, as the skin becomes more naturally lubricated and the burn scars settle down, the itchiness will stop. In the meantime, here are some tips to cope with the itching problem:

- Cleanse with lukewarm, not hot, water.
- Maintain lightly lubricated skin at all times.
- Add bath oil to a bath or apply after a shower.
- Avoid warm places.
- Apply cool towels to areas that are itching.
- If recommended, wear pressure garments.
- Wear loose, 100% cotton clothing next to the affected skin.
- If possible, adjust humidity and temperature in your home to avoid excessive dryness.
- Avoid scratching or rubbing the itchy area.

If you do have to scratch, wear gloves or at least use the pads of your fingers. Never scratch with your fingernails; this can cause damage to the delicate, healing skin.

If you live in an extremely dry or hot climate, such as in the mountains or desert, consider purchasing an air conditioner and limit your time outdoors.

New sensitivity to heat and cold

Your newly-healing skin will be thinner than before your injury and you may experience greater sensitivity to heat and cold. It is possible you may feel a tingling or numbing sensation in your hands and feet in cold weather, or find you sweat more from uninjured areas of your body when it is warm. Over time, as the long healing process takes place, these feelings should diminish.

The key to coping with these unusual feelings is to adjust your activities and clothing in line with your tolerance and reactions.

Avoiding overexposure to sunlight

Your newly-healed skin will be sensitive to sunlight, particularly for the first six months after healing. There are three major problems when you expose your healing skin to sunlight:

- You can sunburn very quickly.
- Healed burn areas can turn permanently dark brown.
- The sun withdraws much-needed moisture from your skin.

The most important advice here is to avoid direct sunlight at all times. In fact, with a burn injury, it is advisable to stay out of direct sunlight for at least six months. After that time, you may expose yourself to direct sunlight for very short periods, as frequently as possible. Protect your injured skin with light-coloured cotton clothing. If your face and neck were subject to burn injury, wear a large-brimmed hat and sunglasses. Also, apply total sunblocks to protect your skin from the sun's rays. You can ask your pharmacist for sunblocks containing high levels of para-aminobenzoic acids, or PABA, to ensure the greatest protection possible. Remember, however, that a sunblock does not totally block the sun's rays – it only increases the time required for the sun's rays to take effect.

Dealing with blisters

It is common for pressure or friction exerted against the sensitive areas of healed skin to cause blisters to develop. Over time, as your skin becomes thicker, blisters will develop less frequently. Do not deliberately puncture your blisters. If they should burst, keep them clean and open to the air to promote healing. If you are wearing pressure garments, small blisters or areas of skin breakdown can be protected with a small piece of plastic kitchen wrap, such as Saran™ Wrap. If the open area is large and does not heal within a week, stop wearing pressure garments temporarily and contact your physician or burn team as soon as possible.

Dealing with skin discolouration

The good news is that, over a period of less than two years, most discolouration will fade. Areas of deeper burns may not return to exactly the same colour as before the burn injury, but you will notice improvements.

The range of discolouration can vary from pale pink to deep purple. This colour is influenced by temperature, the level of your activities, whether you are sitting or standing, if your arms are hanging down by your sides for prolonged periods of time, and your schedule for wearing pressure garments.

As long as you have some form of redness, the newly healed skin will be vulnerable to a number of problems, such as blistering, which are related to fragile skin. You are advised to keep to the skin care recommendations for the period of time it takes for things to settle down.

Once your healed skin is past the blistering stage, you may be interested in paramedical cosmetic camouflage. Both men and women can learn to use these cosmetics that are specially blended for people recovering from burns. These cosmetics, which have high levels of pigment, are usually waterproof, and can be blended to match the colour of your adjacent, uninjured skin. If you are interested in learning more, ask your burn team.

Here are some brands highly recommended by the burn teams we spoke to:

- Dermacolor
- Dermage
- Eva Bouchard®
- Dermablend®
- Covermark®
- Corrective Concepts®
- Cover FX®

Managing your maturing scar

This aspect of skin care is a critical and specialized topic that will require your vigilance and discipline to ensure a successful outcome. Once your burn has healed, only the first stage of recovery is completed. The second and longer stage involves the management of the maturing burn scars.

Over time, you will notice that your flat, smooth burn is not only becoming redder, but is increasingly raised and tight as well. These changes are normal for a maturing burn scar and will continue to occur unless an equal and opposing force is applied.

Your occupational therapist and burn physician may recommend one or more of the following pressure products: a tensor bandage; an elastic tubular support bandage called a Tubigrip®; Isotoner® Gloves, or Coban® Self-Adherent Wrap. There are also rigid face masks and custom-made pressure garments.

To be effective, all products must be worn continuously, for 23 ½ hours a day, taken off only for bathing or showering. It's necessary to do this for a year to a year and a half, or until the redness and elevation of your scars have settled. This sounds like a long time but it's a necessary part of treatment. After the 12 to 18 months, you will be glad you persevered.

It is important to note that these pressure products are not effective once your scars are mature. So be disciplined and stick to your schedule for wearing these products during this optimal period of recovery.

Custom-made garments

When burn scars are either extensive or thickening and will not respond to alternative methods of pressure, your physician may prescribe custom-made garments for you. You may be measured for these garments in the hospital before being discharged or in the burn clinic during one of your follow-up visits. Again, you must wear these garments at all times; it is recommended that your purchase two sets so that one is available while the other is being laundered.

It takes time to get used to these garments, because maturing burn scars are fragile. Your burn team will advise you how to use them. For example, you may wear them for just one or two hours the first day, five or six hours the second day, six to twelve hours the third day, and so on. By the end of the first week the garments should be worn for the full 23 ½ hours a day.

Changing burn dressings at home

You or one of your family members may be required to change a dressing at home. This will probably occur after you have had many dressing changes carried out at the hospital. You should also have received careful instructions from the burn team or have received home care nursing services for a time.

The most important simple factor is to ensure that everything that touches the wound is clean.

What you need

- A work area with a clean, flat surface in a warm room
- A bathtub, sink or basin
- An abrasive cleaner
- Mild soap
- Scissors
- A clean, soft washcloth and a towel

- A small, clean cup
- A wooden applicator
- The recommended topical ointment
- Dressings and gauze bandages

What to do

- Place all the equipment on the work surface.
- Scrub the tub, sink, or basin with cleanser and rinse thoroughly.
- Wash hands thoroughly with soap and water; dry them on a towel.
- Fill the tub, sink, or basin with lukewarm water; mild soap may be added.
- Remove the outer dressing by cutting it off with scissors. Do not pull the dressing off if it is sticking to the wound; instead, soak it in the tub.
- Soak the wound in lukewarm water for 10 to 15 minutes.
- Gently wash the burned area with the washcloth, removing old cream, dried blood and loose skin.
- Using the cup, rinse the wound with clear water.
- Using clean fingers or the wooden applicator, cover the wound with a topical agent or ointment.

Cover the topical agent or ointment with a gauze dressing, taking care not to touch the sides of the dressing that will come into contact with the wound. Wrap snugly with 6 to 7 layers of bandage.

Wash the tub, sink or basin with a cleanser and then rinse thoroughly.

Launder the washcloth and towel so that they will be ready to use again within 24 hours.

Nutrition

In the early stages of your burn injury, your body needs lots of calories and high amounts of protein to provide the energy and building blocks to help your skin recover. Thus, your dietician will provide a diet high in calories and protein throughout the critical period of your injury.

As you recover from your burn injury, your nutritional requirements decrease. Consequently, on leaving the hospital, you no longer require these rich diets. You should evolve back into regular meal planning with one important consideration: keep to a nutritious meal plan.

Proper rehabilitation requires that you have all the important food groups as well as vitamins and minerals. Your daily food choices should include selections from each of the four food groups in the standard food guide, referenced at the back of this book.

In summary, you need the following every day:

- Meat and meat alternatives, for protein, vitamins and minerals vital for skin build-up.
- Milk and milk products, for protein and calcium.
- Breads and cereals, for carbohydrate energy.
- Fruits and vegetables, for vitamins and minerals essential for skin, hair and muscle function.
- Fluids, such as water, orange juice and milk. Use your thirst as an indicator of your fluid needs.

If ever you feel you need guidance or counseling on your dietary needs, contact either your dietician from the hospital or your family physician who can direct you to a local dietician for assistance.

Exercise

Throughout your stay in the hospital, you will probably be on a program of exercises to help maintain your range of motion, strength and endurance. It is important to continue this program after your discharge. Your physical and occupational therapists will likely confirm this and provide you with a suggested exercise program to further your recovery.

Even though you may be completely recovered in terms of being as mobile as you should be, you may feel stiffness and slight pulling in your joints after a period of inactivity or sleep. Exercise will help decrease this stiffness and help you maintain your mobility and avoid contractures.

More often than not, burn survivors have limited movement in some joints at the time of discharge from the hospital. It may be necessary to continue seeing a physical therapist and/or occupational therapist. You may be referred to a rehabilitation hospital when you leave the burn centre or you may be scheduled to visit the rehabilitation medicine department at your local hospital.

It's important to have realistic expectations – aim for a gradual recovery. You cannot recover overnight; it takes time, patience and sustained effort. When you first come home, you'll probably feel more tired than usual. Over time, your energy will return and you'll be able to do more. Try to develop' regular exercise routines and feel good about what you're able to accomplish.

Your occupational therapist may advise you to use splints to help in the recovery process. There are two types:

1. Serial or static splints

These are used following your range of motion (ROM) exercises in order to maintain a joint at the maximum range achieved. These splints may be used at rest or throughout the night in order to apply a constant stretch to tight joints.

2. Dynamic splints

These apply a direct and opposing force to reverse any contracture which may already be present. Since these splints apply a strong stretch force to contracted joints, they should only be worn for up to two hours at a time, three times a day.

Splints may be necessary for up to 18 months or until your joints have reached a maximum range of motion.

Frequently asked questions

Will my burned skin return to its natural colour?

Each person heals differently. Some areas of your burned skin may remain darker or lighter than normal for varying periods of time. It takes about two years for most of the improvements to take place.

If I get a scratch or cut on my healed burn, what should I do?

Although your healed skin is very fragile, it will heal normally with time. You should not be too concerned but you should care for the skin, always keeping it moist.

Some of the skin where I was burned is now so tight and tough. Will it ever be soft again?

Yes. Over a two-year period, it will gradually soften with stretching, using a moisturizer and wearing your pressure garments.

If I am having problems with my splints, do I have to wait until my next scheduled visit?

No. You should contact your occupational therapist as soon as possible to arrange an appointment.

How often do I wash my pressure garments?

Daily, when you take a shower or bath.

Should I wear my pressure garments when bathing or swimming?

No. Once a day, you can take your garments off for a short period of time, a half hour for bathing or swimming.

Section 4:
How To Prevent a
Fire in Your Home

In the kitchen

Unplug kettles, frying pans and other appliances when not in use.

Remove pans of cooking oils and fats from the stove when not in use (you could turn on the wrong burner).

Do not hang cloths over the stove to dry (they may fall on the burner).

Keep matches out of reach of children. Use only safety matches.

Have an approved fire extinguisher nearby for grease fires.

In the living room

Provide fire screens for fireplaces as sparks can easily start a fire.

When lighting a fire, never leave it unattended until all the safety precautions are in place.

Provide sufficient electrical outlets for your needs. Do not use extension cords.

Provide deep substantial ashtrays for smokers. Make sure the contents are placed in a metal container or flushed down the toilet before going to bed.

If you are installing a wood or coal stove, fireplace or solid fuel furnace, you should make sure the installation is certified and the products meets the requirements of major certifying agencies. Check this out before making your purchase.

In the bedroom

Never smoke in bed. Many people are killed in fires as a result of bedding becoming ignited from a cigarette in the hands of a sleepy person.

In the basement and the attic

Remove all combustibles and flammables from the basement and attic areas. These could provide fuel to a fire once started and even make it easier for a fire to start.

Make sure a qualified service man checks out and cleans your furnace once a year. As well, the chimney and flue connections should be checked for leaks.

Remove oversized fuses. A 15-ampere fuse is required for regular domestic circuits.

Have your wiring checked periodically by a qualified electrician.

Using smoke detectors

The majority of fire-related deaths occur from the smoke of a fire which contain gases, i.e. carbon monoxide, that can kill you. Consequently, it is essential to use smoke detectors in your home because you can be alerted to the danger in the early stages of a fire.

Powering detectors

Smoke detectors obtain their power from batteries, the household electric current or both. Instead of sound, light signals are available for the hard of hearing. The smoke detector you buy should be listed by a recognized testing laboratory.

If you are using batteries for a smoke detector, make sure you replace them once a year. All certified battery-operated alarms are required to sound a trouble signal when the batteries need to be replaced. These signals last around seven days. So if you are away from home for a long period of time you should check the batteries on your return. Smoke detectors that operate from a household electrical current can be powered by being directly wired into the electric system or by an electrical cord to a plug. In the latter case, be sure there is no on/off switch for that plug because it could be accidentally turned off.

Location of detectors

A critical area that can be isolated from the rest of the house is the basement, especially with the entrance door firmly closed. Statistically, basements account for a significant number of fires. For this reason you should always place a smoke detector at the head of the stairs leading down to the basement.

A smoke detector is also recommended at the head of each stairway leading to an occupied area; this will be well located for bedroom areas, where you need to hear and be awakened in the event of a fire.

False alarms can be irritating and a nuisance. Do not disconnect or cover up the alarm; instead move it to a better location.

Maintenance of smoke detectors

Smoke alarms should be cleaned as recommended by the manufacturer. Make sure you read the instructions thoroughly and make a mental note or a note in your diary when to attend to the detector.

Fire extinguishers

These are used primarily to prevent small fires from becoming large fires. Their presence in your home can be a vital factor in saving lives and minimizing damage. Place fire extinguishers in readily available places that everybody is aware of. Make sure that everybody knows how to use them.

Planning to evacuate your home

You may think it's not important now, but if your house catches fire, you will be extremely glad you planned escape routes for all family members.

You should conduct a fire drill with all family members ensuring that everybody knows :

a) Two ways out of every bedroom.

b) Escape routes for each room in your home.

c) Make sure babysitters, visiting family members and your family know the drill.

d) Decide in advance who will help babies, the elderly and persons with disabilities.

e) Windows are usually an alternative exit. Be sure storm windows and screens can be removed easily from the inside and are big enough to crawl through.

f) If a window leads to a porch or garage roof, that's helpful. If not, an escape ladder r knotted rope should be available.

g) Make sure everybody knows how to break a window effectively, using a heavy object but shielding the face from flying glass and removing jagged edges with a chair leg or shoe.

h) The phone number for the local fire hall — post it next to every telephone.

When fire strikes

When fire is detected, shout to warn the other occupants. Don't wait to get dressed: grab your shoes and a blanket, if they're available. Have a neighbour call the fire department if you don't have time to do so.

Never open a door without checking it for heat and looking for smoke leaking around the edges of the door. If the door is warm, leave it closed and go out through an alternative exit like a window. Place bed linen or clothing around the edges of the door to prevent smoke entering the room.

Don't risk serious injury by jumping from a high window. Open the window a little and sit on the floor to get fresh air or wait on a balcony for rescue. Hang out a sheet to show rescuers your location. Place bedding on the cracks to keep the smoke out.

Smoke, heat and deadly gases coming up from below to the upper levels can be lethal. It can almost act like a chimney in the middle of your home. If you cannot leave an upper room by a window, close the door and wait by an open window for rescue.

When trying to escape, even if the door feels cool, brace your body against it. Open it an inch, but be ready to shut it if you feel the pressure of a hot draft on your hand. If you do decide to leave the house, cover your mouth and nose with a wet cloth. If there is heavy smoke between you and your exit, get down and crawl — there is usually better air near the ground.

When trying to escape it is best to keep calm and do not panic. You can practice your exit with your eyes closed as if there is thick smoke.

If heat and smoke have entered the room, remember that heat and deadly gases rise. Tie a heavy cloth around your nose and mouth. Roll out of bed and crawl to the window. Make sure the door is shut before you open the window. A draft could fan a fire, cutting off your escape.

Meet at a prearranged place to check who is present. Never go back into a burning building. Be especially watchful of children who may go back into burning buildings to rescue pets or personal possessions.

Seek medical attention as soon as possible.

If you live in a high rise apartment

If the fire is in your suite:

- Alert everybody who is the suite.
- Everybody should leave the suite, closing the door but making sure it is unlocked.
- Sound the fire alarm in the corridor.
- Call the fire department, giving your street address, floor and apartment number.
- Leave your floor by the nearest exit stairway, closing the door behind you to prevent the spread of smoke and heat.
- Never use the elevators. Heat can activate some elevator call buttons sending the elevator to the fire floor itself, where dense smoke may interfere with the elevator's light sensitive eye, preventing the doors from closing. Another potential problem is the water from the fire fighting operations may short out the central switch, causing the elevator to stop and leaving you trapped within the elevator.

If the fire is within your building:

- Call the fire department immediately, giving all the necessary details. Never assume this has already been done.
- Unplug all appliances.

When you evacuate:

Be prepared for heavy smoke and heat. If time allows, put on shoes and a heavy coat for protection. Cover your nose and mouth with a wet cloth.

Test the surfaces of all the doors before opening. If the door or the knob feels hot, deadly heat and gases may have already filled the corridor. Even if the door is cool, brace yourself against the door and open it slightly. If you feel air pressure or a hot draft, close the door quickly. Remain in your suite.

If the corridor is clear, close the suite door behind you and leave the building via the nearest stairway, closing the door after you.

Do not use elevators.

If you encounter smoke or fire in your descent, use another exit. If an alternative exit cannot be reached safely, either return to your suite or seek refuge in a neighbor's apartment.

If you remain in your apartment, use wet towels or sheets to seal cracks, mail slots, etc. If smoke begins to seep through the central air conditioning outlets, plug them as well.

Move to the balcony, or the most protected room and open a window.

If the smoke enters a room, crouch low. If the apartment fills with smoke, go to the balcony. Signal your position by waving a white sheet. Wait to be rescued.

Preventing a fire in an apartment

Keep to the same principles of prevention already mentioned covering homes where appropriate.

Do not put flammable liquids, aerosol cans or burning material down garbage chutes or force anything into chutes which may cause blockages.

It is wise not to use barbeques on balconies due to limited space and the hazards created by the use of starter fluids.

In storage and locker rooms, keep the area tidy, do not store flammable liquids and do not use matches or candles to look for objects in dark lockers.

Internet Sites for Burn Survivors

The Phoenix Society –
http://www.phoenix-society.org

Burn Survivors Throughout the World -
http://www.burnsurvivorsttw.org

Injury related websites –
NCIPC
http:// www.cdc.gov/ncipc/injweb/websites.htm

Canadian Burn Survivors
http://www.canmadianburnsurvivors.ca *

American Burn Association
http://www.ameriburn.org *

*These sites have lists of all the burn centers throughout North America

Other Sites You May want to Google:

- Burn centers, foundations and injury prevention sites
- Alberta Burn Rehabilitation Centre
- Alisa Ann Ruch Burn Foundation
- Arizona Burn Center at Maricopa Medical Center
- British Columbia Professional Firefighters Burn Fund
- Burn Prevention Foundation
- Georgia Firefighters Burn Foundation
- Joseph M. Still Burn Center at Doctors Hospital of Augusta
- International burn Foundation
- Loyola University Health System Burn Center, Maywood Illinois
- National SAFE kids Campaign
- North Carolina Jaycee Burn Center/ UNC Hospitals
- St. Barnabas Burn Foundation
- Shriners Hospital for Children
- The Trauma Foundation
- University of California San Diego Burn Center
- University of Utah Hospital Burn Center
- University of Michigan Burn Center
- University of Washington Burn Center / Harborview, Seattle, WA
- University of Washington Burn InjuryRehabiliatation Model System